Human Ovary
Basic and Clinical Physiology

Akmal El-Mazny

Copyright © 2017 Akmal El-Mazny

All rights reserved.

CreateSpace, Charleston SC, USA

ISBN-13: 978-1541277748
ISBN-10: 1541277740

Contents

	Page
Introduction	1
Overview	2
Physiology of Ovulation	5
– Hormonal Control	5
– Ovarian Cycle	13
– Oocyte Development	19
Ovarian Factors of Infertility	24
Hypergonadotropic Hypogonadism	27
Hypogonadotropic Hypogonadism	28
Polycystic Ovary Syndrome	29
Prolactin Disorders	33
Chromosomal Abnormalities	34
Assessment of Ovulation	36
Ovarian Reserve	37
Ovarian Stimulation	38
– Oral Agents	38
– Gonadotropins	44
– Gonadotropin Releasing Hormone	47
Ovarian Stimulation for IVF	53
– Long Protocol	57
– Short and Ultrashort Protocols	58
– Antagonist Protocol	59
Ovarian Hyperstimulation Syndrome	64
References	68

INTRODUCTION

The female reproductive system is a complicated but fascinating subject; it has the capability to function intimately with nearly every other body system for the purpose of reproduction.

The female reproductive system consists of the hypothalamic-pituitary unit, the ovaries, and the reproductive tract.

The functions of the ovaries are to produce oocytes, for sexual reproduction, and produce hormones that regulate reproductive function and secondary sex characteristics.

Abnormalities in the physiologic function of the ovary affect the development of oocytes and potential fertility.

This book provides a comprehensive review of the physiology specific to the ovary, emphasizing abnormalities affecting its function and the mechanisms behind treatment.

I hope this book will enhance your knowledge of the basic and clinical physiology of the ovary, and that you will be able to apply this information to your practice.

OVERVIEW

The ovaries are paired organs located on either side of the uterus within the mesovarium portion of the broad ligament below the uterine tubes.

At birth, a female has approximately 1-2 million eggs, but only 300 of these eggs ever mature and are released for the purpose of fertilization.

The ovaries are small and oval-shaped, exhibit a grayish color, and have an uneven surface.

The actual size of an ovary depends on a woman's age and hormonal status; the ovaries are approximately 3-5 cm in length during childbearing years and become much smaller and atrophic once menopause occurs.

A cross-section of the ovary reveals many cystic structures that vary in size representing ovarian follicles at different stages of development and degeneration.

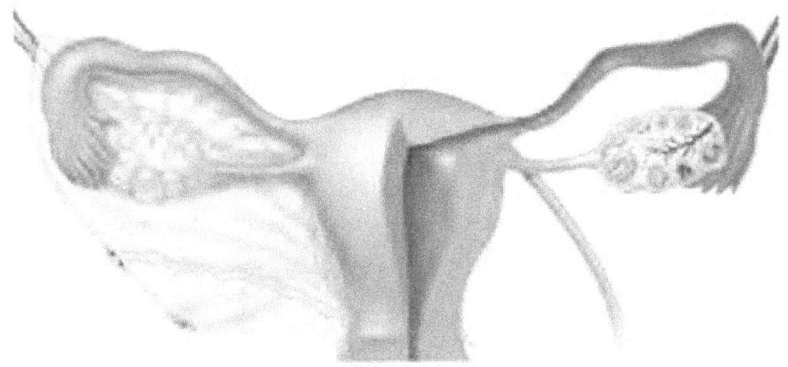

Gross Anatomy of the Ovaries

Several ligaments support the ovary:

– The ovarian ligament connects the uterus and ovary.

– The posterior portion of the broad ligament forms the mesovarium, which supports the ovary and houses the vascular supply.

– The suspensory (infundibular) ligament of the ovary, a peritoneal fold overlying the ovarian vessels, attaches the ovary to the pelvic side wall.

Blood supply to the ovary is via the ovarian artery; both right and left ovarian arteries originate directly from the descending aorta at the level of the L2 vertebra, and enter the ovary at the hilum.

The left ovarian vein drains into the left renal vein, and the right ovarian vein empties directly into the inferior vena cava.

Lymphatic drainage of the ovary is primarily to the lateral aortic nodes; however, the iliac nodes may also be involved.

Nerve supply to the ovaries, through the ovarian, hypogastric, and aortic plexuses, run with the vasculature within the suspensory ligament of the ovary entering the ovary at the hilum.

Microscopic Anatomy of the Ovary

The ovaries are covered externally by a layer of simple cuboidal epithelium called germinal (ovarian) epithelium.

Beneath this layer is a dense connective tissue capsule (tunica albuginea).

The main body of the ovary is divided into an outer cortex and an inner medulla.

The cortex is dense and granular and contains numerous ovarian follicles in various stages of development.

The medulla is loose connective tissue with abundant blood vessels, lymphatic vessels, and nerve fibers.

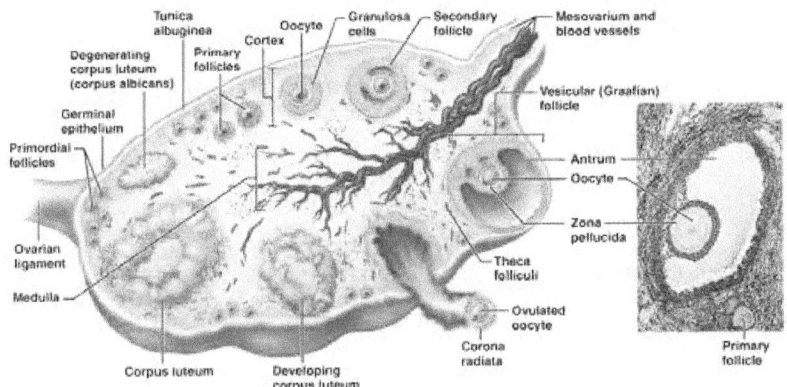

Microscopic Anatomy of the Ovary

Functions of the Ovary

- The ovary cyclically produces gametes; the number of oocytes (germ cells) available is determined during fetal development and continues to decline by either ovulation or atresia until menopause occurs.

- It also cyclically secretes hormones (androgens, estrogens, progestins) that prepare the reproductive tract for oocyte transport, fertilization, implantation and pregnancy, and it controls the hypothalamic-pituitary unit through negative and positive feedback mechanisms.

PHYSIOLOGY OF OVULATION

Hormonal Control

There are four major functional compartments involved in reproduction, each has a specific function: the hypothalamus, the pituitary gland and the ovaries, which compose the hypothalamic-pituitary-ovarian axis; and the hormonally-responsive functional endometrium lining the uterus.

In the presence of low levels of estrogen, the arcuate nucleus of the hypothalamus releases gonadotropin releasing hormone (GnRH).

This hormone signals the anterior pituitary to produce the gonadotropins leutinizing hormone (LH) and follicle-stimulating hormone (FSH).

These gonadotropins in turn induce the development and maturation of ovarian follicles that contain the actual oocytes.

The growing follicles produce increased amounts of estradiol.

This increase in estrogen production develops the endometrium and thins the increasing amounts of cervical mucus.

When the estradiol level reaches an appropriate level, generally when the follicle is mature, the pituitary releases a large amount of LH.

LH surge causes the final maturation of the oocyte and stimulates the event of ovulation.

After the oocyte is released, that is, ovulation occurs, the sac containing the oocyte undergoes metamorphosis with growth of new blood vessels and becomes a functioning gland called the corpus luteum.

The corpus luteum produces progesterone in large amounts and estrogen in smaller amounts; progesterone stabilizes the endometrium and thickens the cervical mucus.

The lifespan of the corpus luteum is about 14 days; if the woman does not conceive, the corpus luteum stops producing progesterone, the endometrium is no longer stable, and menses begin.

The normal menstrual cycle length is 25 to 35 days; this cyclicity is determined by changing sensitivities of the hypothalamic-pituitary unit to estrogens and progestins.

The hypothalamic-pituitary-ovarian axis also involves a negative feedback loop in which gonadal secretions produced in response to pituitary gonadotropins inhibit further secretion of gonadotropins.

The hypothalamic-pituitary-ovarian axis in the female also involves a positive feedback loop in which ovarian estrogen produced in response to pituitary FSH enhances pituitary secretion of LH and FSH.

Female Hormones: Production and Action

Functional Compartment	Location	Hormone or Function
- Hypothalamus	- Arcuate nucleus	- GnRH
- Anterior pituitary	- Gonadotropin	- FSH
		- LH
- Ovary	- Follicle	- Estradiol
	- Corpus luteum	- Progesterone
		- Inhibin
		- Activin
		- Anti-Mullerian hormone
- Uterus	- Endometrium	- Proliferative
		- Secretory
		- Menses

Physiology of Ovulation

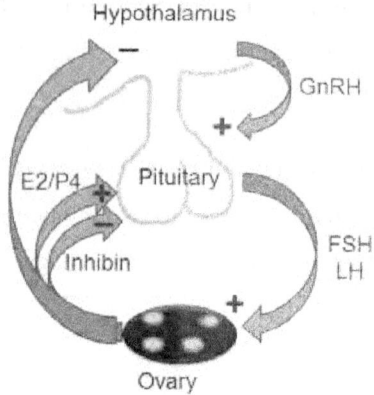

Hypothalamic-Pituitary-Ovarian Axis

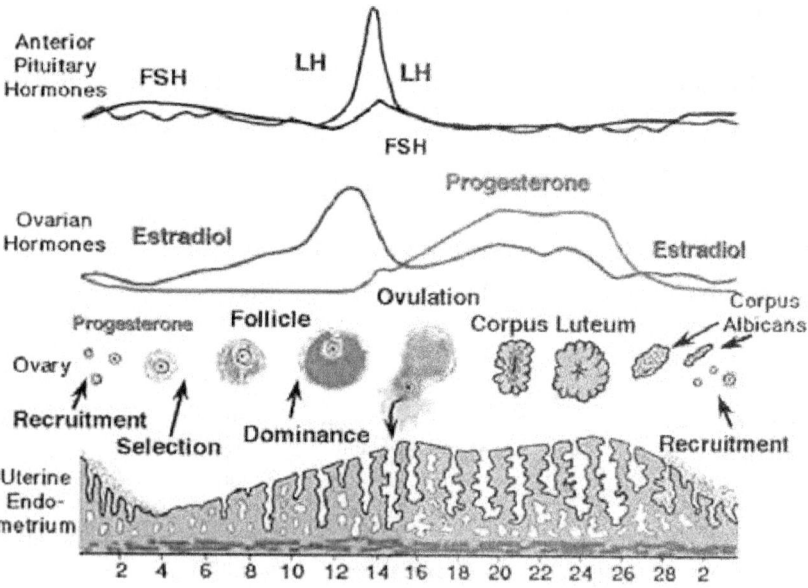

Hormonal Control

Hypothalamus - GnRH

GnRH is synthesized and secreted by neurons in the arcuate nucleus of the hypothalamus and diffuses into the hypothalamic-hypophyseal portal vessels, which transport it to the anterior pituitary gland.

Through pulsatile release, GnRH stimulates the gonadotropes to produce FSH and LH.

The activity of this decapeptide can be modified by changing one or more amino acids; this creates GnRH agonists or antagonists that are often used as adjuncts to infertility and other medical disorders.

Anterior Pituitary - FSH

FSH is a heterodimeric glycoprotein synthesized in gonadotropes in the anterior pituitary.

It has a relatively long half-life in the plasma, normally 3-4 hours; peripheral plasma levels of FSH do not reflect pulsatile GnRH secretion.

FSH stimulates granulosa cells of the ovarian follicle and the luteinized cells of the corpus luteum.

It is considered the critical regulator of follicular development because it is capable of stimulating follicular development by itself.

FSH is suppressed by rising estradiol from the growing follicle; cyclic levels are at their maximum on Day 3 and midcycle surge.

The number of primary follicles which begin to enlarge and respond to FSH is related to the age and total number of oocytes present in the ovary.

Anterior Pituitary - LH

LH is a heterodimeric glycoprotein synthesized in the same gonadotropes in the anterior pituitary as FSH.

LH has a shorter plasma half life (about 20 minutes) than FSH, so peripheral plasma levels do reflect the pronounced pulsatile pattern of GnRH secretion.

LH is secreted in a pulsatile manner: in the follicular phase of the female menstrual cycle, the pulse interval is normally 90 min; and in the luteal phase it is about 2 to 3 hours.

LH stimulates mature granulosa cells of the preovulatory follicle and their successor cells, the luteinized cells of the corpus luteum.

LH is capable of maintaining the lifespan of the corpus luteum beyond the normal luteal phase of the menstrual cycle; however, LH is rapidly degraded when administered by injection.

LH has the following stimulatory effects on ovarian cells:

– Increases availability of free cholesterol.

– Stimulates production of androgens in ovarian theca and interstitial cells by increasing enzymes for androgen biosynthesis.

– Increases production of progesterone and estradiol in the corpus luteum.

– Increases plasminogen activator synthesis and secretion in granulosa cells of the preovulatory follicle.

– Stimulates resumption of meiosis in the oocyte at midcycle.

Ovary - Sex Steroids

Although the ovary secretes many steroid hormones including androgens, estrogens and progestins, appear to be among the most important.

Androgens are synthesized in the theca and interstitial cells and are important as substrates for estrogen biosynthesis.

The adrenal glands are the principal source of circulating androgens (dehydroepiandrosterone, androstenedione, and testosterone) in women.

The increase in synthesis of adrenal androgens at puberty (called adrenarche) stimulates the development of axillary, pubic and facial hair.

High levels of androgens suppress progesterone synthesis in granulosa cells.

Although the ovaries and adrenals produce similar quantities of androstenedione and testosterone, most of the ovarian androgens are converted to estrogens in the ovaries and in peripheral tissues.

Most of the testosterone in the plasma of the adult female is formed by peripheral conversion of androstenedione by peripheral 17β-hydroxysteroid dehydrogenase.

Estradiol is considered the most important product of the granulosa cells of the developing follicle; estrone is a less active estrogen than estradiol.

Estradiol concentrations in plasma reach a peak during the late follicular phase, decline after ovulation and then rise again during the luteal phase.

Progesterone is considered the most important product of the corpus luteum.

Ovary - Inhibins

Inhibin is a heterodimeric glycoprotein consisting of an alpha and a beta subunit and is synthesized by granulosa and luteal cells of the ovary.

FSH stimulates granulosa cells to synthesize and secrete inhibin, so that as follicles enlarge, they produce increasing amounts of the hormone.

Inhibin preferentially inhibits synthesis and secretion of FSH but not LH by pituitary gonadotropes (negative feedback), elimination of inhibin results in a rise in FSH secretion.

Inhibin production is low at the beginning of the menstrual cycle, then increases late in the follicular phase and reaches a peak prior to the preovulatory surge of FSH and LH.

After ovulation, inhibin levels decrease slightly, followed by a final rise in the midluteal phase to a level twice that at midcycle.

As the corpus luteum regresses, inhibin levels decline and FSH levels rise with the beginning of the next menstrual cycle.

Ovary - Activins

Activin, a dimeric protein consisting of two of the β subunits of inhibin, is secreted by the ovarian granulosa cells.

Activin amplifies the effect of FSH on granulosa cells in the ovary.

It also increases the synthesis of FSH β subunit in the anterior pituitary.

Activin is synthesized in numerous other tissues, but the role in those tissues is not understood.

Physiology of Ovulation

Neuroendocrine Control

Inhibin, acts on the pituitary to suppress the synthesis and release of FSH, but does not impact LH.

In the follicular phase, estrogen exerts negative feedback by decreasing the pulse amplitude thereby decreasing FSH and LH pulse amplitude.

In the luteal phase, progesterone and testosterone decrease GnRH pulse frequency resulting in decreased FSH and LH pulse frequency.

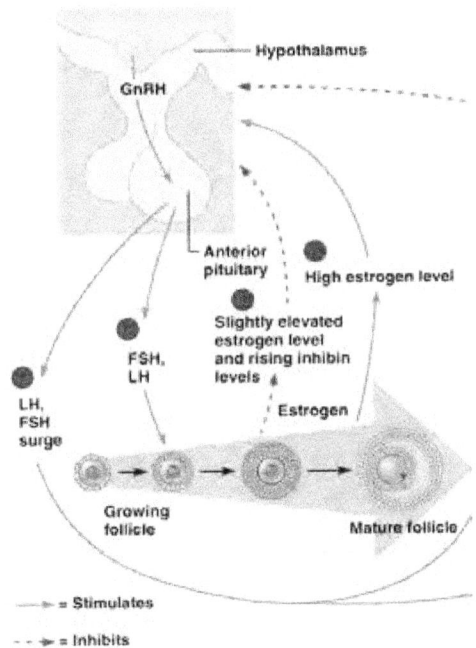

Neuroendocrine Control

Ovarian Cycle

The follicle is the basic functional unit of the ovary.

Each follicle consists of an oocyte surrounded by one or more layers of specialized cells (granulosa, theca) which secrete autocrine, paracrine, and endocrine factors.

The follicle grows under the influence of gonadotropins (FSH, LH) and intraovarian regulators (estradiol, IGF-I, activin).

Development from a primordial follicle to a preovulatory follicle takes three to four menstrual cycles.

Follicular Phase

Primordial Follicle

- Primordial follicles are formed during fetal life and are not believed to require gonadotropins for formation; however, females lacking functional FSH receptors have poorly developed ovaries.

- A primordial follicle consists of an oocyte and a single layer of epithelial cells.

- The oocyte is arrested in the first meiotic prophase.

- During the first cycle of development the oocyte grows to about 100 microns in diameter and the epithelial cells enlarge and become cuboidal granulosa cells; at this point, the oocyte is referred to as the "primary follicle".

- FSH receptors are first detectable on the plasma membrane of granulosa cells.

- The granulosa cells respond to FSH by proliferating faster.

Preantral Follicle

- During the first to second cycles of development, the primary follicle progresses to the preantral stage.

- Oocyte meiosis remains arrested.

- The oocyte completes the first step of meiotic maturation, which includes germinal vesicle breakdown and metaphase I after the mid-cycle LH surge.

- Preantral follicles respond to the midcycle surge of FSH during the second to third cycles of development by growing rapidly; this event is called recruitment.

- All recruited follicles produce sex steroid hormones in amounts proportional to their size and degree of maturation.

- A single follicle, the most mature follicle, becomes dominant.

- The remaining follicles degenerate through a process called atresia.

- The emergence of the single dominant follicle appears to result from the inhibin-induced decline in plasma FSH concentrations.

- Once a dominant follicle is selected, rising serum hormone levels of inhibin and estradiol suppress FSH.

- Local production of estradiol by the dominant follicle amplifies the response to FSH.

- Estradiol synthesis continues to increase exponentially in response to FSH.

Antral Follicle

- Fluid accumulates among the granulosa cells forming a fluid-filled cavity, the antrum.

- After the antrum is formed, the follicle is termed a "secondary follicle".

Preovulatory Follicle

- During the last cycle of development (third or fourth cycle), the dominant follicle attains its maximal size and the theca layer vascularizes; this represents the "Graafian follicle".

- The oocyte (meiosis still arrested) has the capacity to proceed to metaphase II and complete meiotic maturation after fertilization.

- Granulosa cells of immature follicles have few LH receptors so they don't respond to LH at physiological LH concentrations.

- The theca cells (and the interstitial cells) do have LH receptors and they respond to LH.

- One of the actions of FSH on granulosa cells during the follicular phase of the menstrual cycle is to induce LH receptors so that granulosa cells of the preovulatory Graafian follicle become responsive to LH as well as to FSH.

− After the LH/FSH surge prior to ovulation, the granulosa cells initially decrease their LH and FSH receptors and then increase them as the granulosa cells luteinize to become the corpus luteum.

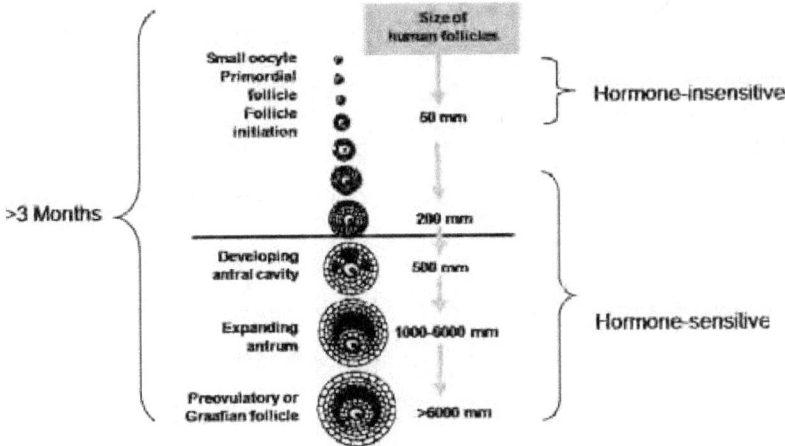

Follicle Development

Ovulation Phase

− LH triggers several processes that culminate in ovulation.

− LH causes a resumption of oocyte meiosis, and metaphase I is completed.

− The first polar body is extruded, and meiosis then halts in metaphase II.

− An increase in follicular pressure, combined with LH-activated breakdown of the follicular wall results in follicular rupture.

− The cumulus-oocyte complex is ovulated 34-36 hours after the onset of the LH surge, and the remaining granulosa and theca cells luteinize.

Luteal Phase

- After ovulation the follicular cells luteinize and form the corpus luteum (literally, yellow body).

- They acquire the capacity to secrete progesterone, and lipid droplets accumulate in the cells.

- If the oocyte is fertilized and implants in the endometrium, the corpus luteum remains active and secretes progesterone in large amounts and estradiol in smaller amounts.

- Progesterone from the corpus luteum prepares the endometrium for implantation and maintains the fetal-placental unit during the first half of the first trimester of pregnancy.

- The corpus luteum requires low levels of LH for continued function.

- LH stimulates the production of progesterone and estradiol, and FSH stimulates the production of estradiol only.

- If fertilization and implantation do not occur, the corpus luteum degenerates (called luteolysis), and progesterone declines within 10 days after ovulation.

- Unlike the variable length of the follicular phase of the menstrual cycle, the luteal phase has a lifespan of about 14 days; this lifespan is due to the fairly consistent lifespan of the corpus luteum.

- However, if pregnancy occurs, the corpus luteum is rescued by hCG that is produced by the implanted trophoblasts.

—LH and hCG are similar in structure; hCG may be thought of as long acting LH.

—In clinical situations hCG injections are used to act like LH, particularly to induce ovulation or stimulate luteal progesterone production.

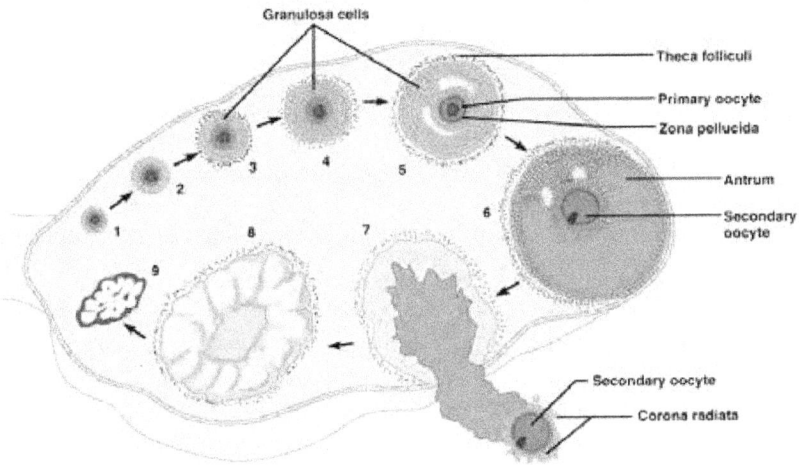

Ovarian Cycle

Oocyte Development

The ovaries and germ cells (which develop into oocytes) form during the first few weeks of embryonic life.

These germ cells rapidly divide by a process called mitosis, in which each new daughter cell contains the same number of chromosomes as the parent cell.

During the first trimester of embryonic growth, these preoocyte cells are called oogonium (plural: oogonia).

During the second trimester of life, the 46 chromosomes start to replicate through the process of meiosis but remain within the cell.

At this stage of meiosis, the cell is called a primary oocyte (primitive ovum not yet fully developed).

At this point, further chromosome separation and oocyte development are arrested until after puberty.

These primary oocytes are surrounded by a layer of epithelium that gives rise to the primordial follicles.

About 1700 germ cells are present before migration to the genital ridge begins.

However, these multiply during the process of migration, reaching a peak of 7 million oocytes at midgestation.

The primordial germ cells increase in size early in their development and become oogonia.

The oocytes remain fertile for only 15-18 hours after ovulation while sperm are motile for 24 hours to several days after ejaculation.

When a sperm encounters the zona pellucida, it undergoes an acrosome reaction; this breaks down the acrosomal membrane.

The sperm head membrane binds to the sperm receptor, which is followed by fusion with the oolemma.

Microvilli on the oocyte surface surround the sperm head and the oocyte undergoes the cortical reaction (release of cortical granules).

The zona pellucida hardens and no other sperm can penetrate the oolemma.

The oocyte nucleus completes maturation to yield the female pronucleus and the second polar body; the sperm nucleus forms the male pronucleus.

The corona radiata is the layer of granulosa cells surrounding the oocyte; the zona pellucida is an extracellular layer of proteins surrounding the oocyte.

Egg Activation

The process of egg activation occurs after fertilization, and involves the completion of the second meiotic division and initiation of embryonic development.

Mitosis begins and there are changes in maternal messenger ribonucleic acids and protein synthesis.

Exocytosis of cortical granules blocks polyspermy and cytoskeletal rearrangement occurs.

Physiology of Ovulation

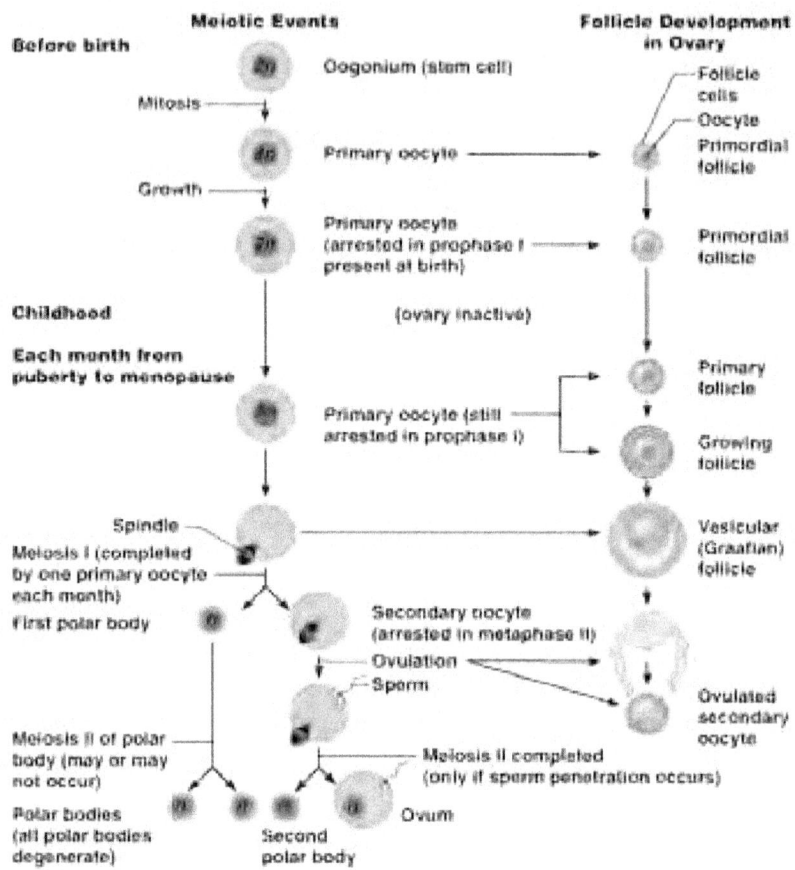

Oocyte Development

OVARIAN FACTORS OF INFERTILITY

Oogenesis occurs in the ovary from the first trimester of embryonic life and is completed by 28-30 weeks of gestation.

By then, approximately 7 million oocytes are arrested at the prophase stage of the first meiosis division.

Subsequently, the number of oocytes decreases because of a continuous process of atresia.

At birth, the pool of oocytes is reduced to approximately 2 million.

By menarche, approximately 500,000 oocytes are present.

Those oocytes are used throughout the reproductive years until menopause.

The ovulatory process is initiated once the hypothalamus-pituitary-ovarian axis matures and FSH and LH, under the regulation of GnRH, acquire their normal secretory patterns.

From the cohort of follicles available each month, only a single oocyte is selected, establishes dominance, and develops to the preovulatory stage.

During follicular development, the granulosa cells secrete increasing amounts of E_2, initially down-regulating the secretion of FSH.

Later, through a positive feedback mechanism, E_2 generates the LH surge that triggers the ovulatory process, induces the resumption of meiosis by the oocyte, and stimulates the formation of the corpus luteum and subsequent progesterone secretion.

Ovulatory dysfunction is defined as an alteration in the frequency and duration of the menstrual cycle.

Failure to ovulate is the most common infertility problem.

Absence of ovulation can be associated with primary amenorrhea, secondary amenorrhea, or oligomenorrhea.

Structural entities associated with primary amenorrhea include congenital absence of the uterus, vagina, or hymen (cryptomenorrhea).

Secondary amenorrhea is the absence of menses for more than 6 months in a woman who has previously menstruated.

In the absence of pregnancy, this condition is related to dysfunction of the endocrine system and can be related to thyroid, adrenal, and pituitary disorders, including tumors.

One common cause of secondary amenorrhea is premature ovarian failure, which is the loss of ovarian function by the age of 40.

Oligomenorrhea is a dysfunction of the hypothalamus-pituitary-ovarian axis and is the most common ovulatory disorder associated with infertility.

Patients with this disorder present with a history of irregular menstrual cycles that fluctuate from 35 days to 2-5 months, sometimes associated with a history of dysfunctional uterine bleeding or prolonged periods of breakthrough bleeding.

Patients may have symptoms of hyperandrogenism, acne, hirsutism, and baldness; obesity is frequently associated and aggravates the prognosis.

Although these patients are not sterile, their fertility is decreased, and the obstetrical outcome is generally poor because of an increased risk of pregnancy loss.

Causes of Ovulatory Infertility

– Hypergonadotropic hypogonadism.

– Hypogonadotropic hypogonadism.

– Polycystic ovary syndrome.

– Prolactin disorders.

– Chromosomal abnormalities.

HYPERGONADOTROPIC HYPOGONADISM

Hypergonadotropic hypogonadism is often related to gonadal development failure, as in Turner syndrome, where the karyotype 45,X indicates an absence of an X chromosome.

These patients present with sexual infantilism associated with short stature, webbed neck, and cubitus valgus.

Streak gonads replace their ovaries, but they have a small uterus and normal fallopian tubes and vagina.

This condition is associated with elevated FSH and LH levels and low estrogen levels.

Other chromosomal abnormalities include 46,XX, which is associated with partial deletions of the short or long arm of one of the X chromosomes, and mosaicism (eg, X/XXX; X/XX/XXX; pure gonadal dysgenesis; 46,XX; 46,XY).

Hypergonadotropic hypogonadism resulting in primary amenorrhea can also be seen in patients with a history of being treated with certain alkylating chemotherapy or pelvic radiation.

Chronic disease conditions, high levels of stress, and starvation or malnutrition are other possible etiologies.

HYPOGONADOTROPIC HYPOGONADISM

Hypogonadotropic hypogonadism refers to suppression of GnRH pulsatility from the hypothalamus, resulting in lack of production of FSH and LH from the pituitary and lack of production of ovarian hormones.

Causes of hypogonadotropic hypogonadism include eating disorders, such as anorexia, bulimia, and disordered eating.

Extreme exercise, is also associated with hypothalamic suppression, as are hyperprolactinemia and hypothyroidism.

CNS lesions, such as craniopharyngioma, can lead to hypogonadotropic hypogonadism.

Kallmann syndrome is caused by failure of the GnRH neurons to migrate during fetal development and is associated with anosmia (inability to smell) and primary amenorrhea.

Hormonal assessment reveals FSH and LH in the low-normal range or very suppressed, less than 3 mIU/mL; estradiol is also suppressed to less than 30 pg/mL.

Longstanding hypogonadotropic hypogonadism is associated with low bone density due to prolonged hypoestrogenism.

Treatment is based on correcting the underlying pathology, treating eating disorders, central nervous system lesions, etc.

If hypogonadotropic hypogonadism persists, then treatment involves the use of gonadotropins to induce ovulation.

POLYCYSTIC OVARY SYNDROME

Polycystic ovary syndrome (PCOS) is the most common endocrinopathy in women.

It has been shown to occur in 4 to 6% of reproductive-aged women, though the prevalence has been reported to be as high as 10%.

It is also considered the single most common cause of infertility due to anovulation.

Diagnostic criteria for PCOS have been defined in the Rotterdam Criteria published in 2003.

Two out of the following three criteria are necessary:

– Oligoovulation or anovulation;

– Clinical and/or biochemical evidence of hyperandrogenism, such as hirsutism, acne, male-pattern baldness on exam or laboratory evaluation demonstrating elevated total testosterone, or free testosterone; and

– Polycystic ovaries demonstrated on ultrasound.

Physical examination typically reveals excess male-pattern hair growth, predominantly in the midline.

However, ethnic differences in hair growth exist and must be taking into consideration.

Acne may be the only sign of hyperandrogenism in teenagers and Asian women.

Acanthosis nigricans is a raised, velvety hyperpigmentation of the skin seen on the dorsal surface of the neck and intertriginous areas, and is a marker of insulin resistance.

Obesity is seen in 50-75% of women with PCOS; however, many women with PCOS are thin.

Health consequences seen in women with PCOS include diabetes, obesity, heart disease, dyslipidemia, hypertension, endometrial hyperplasia, and infertility.

Laboratory assessment includes TSH, prolactin, FSH and estradiol, and 17-hydroxyprogesterone levels.

A total testosterone level is helpful to distinguish a tumor, but it is often normal or only slightly elevated in PCOS.

Free testosterone assay is imprecise, and is therefore often not recommended.

DHEAS is produced primarily by the adrenal gland and testing is not recommended unless there is concern about an adrenal tumor.

DHEAS is elevated in only 25% of women with PCOS.

LH/FSH ratio is only elevated (more than 2-fold) in 50-60% of women with PCOS and is non-diagnostic, and therefore it is not recommended.

Ultrasound criteria to diagnose PCOS include:

– The presence of more than 12 follicles of 2 to 9 mm in diameter; and

– Increased ovarian volume of >10 mL^3.

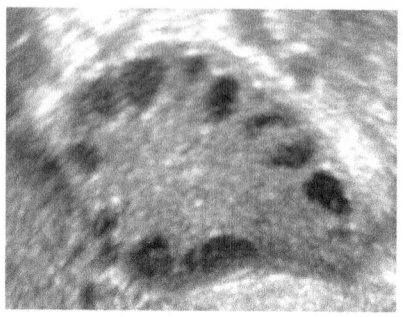
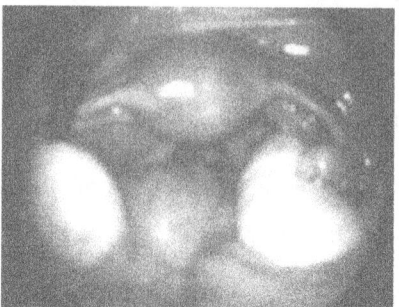

Ultrasonography   **Laparoscopy**

Polycystic Ovary Syndrome (PCOS)

There are multiple treatments available for women with PCOS desiring to conceive.

Weight loss for obese women is important, not only for improving chances of ovulation, but also for reducing the risks during pregnancy.

CC is the first-line drug for treatment of anovulation.

Conception rates per cycle with CC have been reported to be 22%, which is comparable to normal cycle fecundity.

Side effects include hot flushes, moodiness, a 10% rate of twin gestation, and 0.5% rate of triplet gestation.

Metformin is an insulin-sensitizing agent that has been used with off-label indication in the treatment of PCOS.

Studies have shown an increased rate of ovulation with metformin, however, the use of metformin as an adjunct to other therapies in subsets of infertile women with PCOS has yet to be determined.

Gonadotropin therapy for ovulation induction in women with PCOS has been shown to be successful with pregnancy rates of approximately 22%.

OHSS remains a significant concern due multiple follicular development and hypersensitive ovaries.

Laparoscopic ovarian drilling (LOD) involves drilling 3 to 10 holes per ovary at laparoscopy using electrocautery or laser.

In women with PCOS who are resistant to CC, LOD results in ovulation rates of 75 to 85%, which are similar to results seen with adding metformin for CC-resistant women.

Risks of the surgery include ovarian adhesions and ovarian failure if too many holes are drilled.

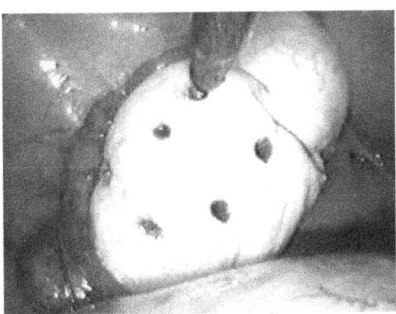

Laparoscopic Ovarian Drilling (LOD)

PROLACTIN DISORDERS

Prolactinomas are the most common pituitary adenoma, accounting for 40%.

Prolactinomas are considered microadenomas if the size is less than 10 mm, and macroadenomas if greater than 10 mm.

Macroadenomas can cause visual symptoms due to their size and compression of the optic chiasm.

Secretion of high levels of prolactin suppresses production of GnRH, leading to decreased FSH and LH, and hypoestrogenism.

Prolactinemia results in galactorrhea and suppresses gonadotropin secretion, leading to amenorrhea.

Presenting symptoms are, therefore, galactorrhea, amenorrhea or both.

Medical therapy involves the use of dopamine agonists to suppress prolactin secretion.

The most commonly used dopamine agonist is bromocriptine.

Cabergoline is a newer option and has fewer side effects.

Once the prolactin level is normalized, ovulation will be restored within a few months.

Macroadenomas can be treated medically, but surgery is often the preferred method for large masses.

CHROMOSOMAL ABNORMALITIES

Chromosomal abnormalities and poor oocyte quality are 2 examples of causes of poor embryonic quality, low implantation rate, increased miscarriage, and low birth rates.

Gene	Encoded Protein	Effect of Deficiency
BMP15	Bone morphogenetic protein 15	Hypergonadotrophic ovarian failure (POF4)
BMPR1B	Bone morphogenetic protein receptor 1B	Ovarian dysfunction, hypergonadotrophic hypogonadism and acromesomelic chondrodysplasia
CBX2; M33	Chromobox protein homolog 2 ; Drosophila polycomb class	Autosomal 46,XY, male-to-female sex reversal
CHD7	Chromodomain-helicase-DNA-binding protein 7	CHARGE syndrome and Kallmann syndrome (KAL5)
DIAPH2	Diaphanous homolog 2	Hypergonadotrophic, premature ovarian failure (POF2A)
FGF8	Fibroblast growth factor 8	Normosmic hypogonadotrophic hypogonadism and Kallmann syndrome (KAL6)
FGFR1	Fibroblast growth factor receptor 1	Kallmann syndrome (KAL2)
HFM1		Primary ovarian failure
FSHR	FSH receptor	Hypergonadotrophic hypogonadism and ovarian hyperstimulation syndrome
FSHB	Follitropin subunit beta	Deficiency of FSH, primary amenorrhoea and infertility
FOXL2	Forkhead box L2	Isolated premature ovarian failure (POF3) associated with BPES type I; FOXL2
FMR1	Fragile X mental retardation	402C --> G mutations associated with human granulosa cell tumours
GNRH1	Gonadotropin releasing hormone	Premature ovarian failure (POF1) associated with premutations
GNRHR	GnRH receptor	Normosmic hypogonadotrophic hypogonadism
KAL1	Kallmann syndrome	Hypogonadotrophic hypogonadism
KISS1R ; GPR54	KISS1 receptor	Hypogonadotrophic hypogonadism and insomnia, X-linked Kallmann syndrome (KAL1)
LHB	Luteinizing hormone beta polypeptide	Hypogonadotrophic hypogonadism

Gene	Encoded Protein	Effect of Deficiency
LHCGR	LH/choriogonadotrophin receptor	Hypogonadism and pseudohermaphroditism
DAX1	Dosage-sensitive sex reversal, adrenal hypoplasia critical region, on chromosome X, gene 1	Hypergonadotrophic hypogonadism (luteinizing hormone resistance)
NR5A1; SF1	Steroidogenic factor 1	X-linked congenital adrenal hypoplasia with hypogonadotrophic hypogonadism; dosage-sensitive male-to-female sex reversal
POF1B	Premature ovarian failure 1B	46,XY male-to-female sex reversal and streak gonads and congenital lipoid adrenal hyperplasia; 46,XX gonadal dysgenesis and 46,XX primary ovarian insufficiency
PROK2	Prokineticin	Hypergonadotrophic, primary amenorrhea (POF2B)
PROKR2	Prokineticin receptor 2	Normosmic hypogonadotrophic hypogonadism and Kallmann syndrome (KAL4)
RSPO1	R-spondin family, member 1	Kallmann syndrome (KAL3)
SRY	Sex-determining region Y	46,XX, female-to-male sex reversal (individuals contain testes)
SOX9	SRY-related HMB-box gene 9	Mutations lead to 46,XY females; translocations lead to 46,XX males
STAG3	Stromal antigen 3	Autosomal 46,XY male-to-female sex reversal (campomelic dysplasia)
TAC3	Tachykinin 3	Premature ovarian failure
TACR3	Tachykinin receptor 3	Normosmic hypogonadotrophic hypogonadism
ZP1	Zona pellucida glycoprotein 1	Normosmic hypogonadotrophic hypogonadism

ASSESSMENT OF OVULATION

Ovulation is usually inferred when a woman reports regular cycles.

If there is doubt, progesterone level greater than 3 ng/mL is indicative of ovulation.

In the absence of pregnancy, progesterone production decreases after that.

Sonographic confirmation of follicle rupture with serial ultrasonography can also be performed.

Correlation with serum estradiol, LH, and progesterone levels are helpful.

Basal body temperature charts can be used to predict ovulation.

A basal body thermometer measures the slight rise in temperature that occurs immediately after ovulation.

However, most patients and physicians prefer to use urinary ovulation predictor kits as they are more accurate and easier to administer.

The LH surge in the serum will last for 36 hours and ovulation occurs 12 hours after the peak of the surge.

Therefore ovulation will occur within 24 hours of detecting the LH surge in urine.

False positives can occur in women who are perimenopausal and in women who have PCOS, as serum LH levels can be elevated in both of these situations.

OVARIAN RESERVE

The level of ovarian reserve and the age of the female partner are the most important prognostic factors in the fertility workup.

Ovarian reserve is most commonly evaluated by checking a cycle day 3 FSH and estradiol level.

Normal ovarian function is indicated when the FSH level is less than 10 mIU/mL and the estradiol level is less than 65 pg/mL.

In cases where the patient is 35 years or older, dynamic ovarian reserve testing may be indicated.

The most common test used is the clomiphene citrate challenge test (CCCT).

Clomiphene citrate (CC) 100 mg by mouth is administered on cycle days 5-9 and a serum FSH level is drawn again on day 10.

An FSH level greater than 10 is associated with decreased fertility and lower pregnancy rates.

Other tests of ovarian reserve include antral follicle counts, ovarian volume, inhibin B, and antimüllerian hormone.

OVARIAN STIMULATION

Ovulation induction is the appropriate treatment for infertile patients who have dysfunction of the hypothalamic-pituitary-ovarian axis.

Oral Agents

Clomiphene Citrate (CC)

The chemical formula for CC is 2-[p-(2-chloro-1,2-difhenylvinyl) phenoxy] triethylamine dihydrogen citrate.

CC is a nonsteroidal selective estrogen receptor modulator (SERM) capable of interacting with estrogen receptor binding proteins in a manner similar to estrogen but in a more prolonged way; therefore, CC behaves similar to an antiestrogen.

CC has been in clinical use since the early 1960s.

Its mechanism of action is still not well understood, but it competes for the estrogen receptor at the hypothalamus, pituitary, and ovarian levels.

Because of the action at the estrogen-receptor level within the hypothalamus, CC alleviates the negative feedback effect exerted by endogenous estrogens.

As a result, CC normalizes the GnRH release; therefore, the secretion of FSH and LH is capable of normalized follicular recruitment, selection, and development to reestablish the normal process of ovulation.

The standard dose of CC is 50 mg PO qd for 5 days, starting on the menstrual cycle day 3-5 or after progestin-induced bleeding.

As an antiestrogen, CC requires that the patient have some circulating estrogen levels; otherwise, the patient will not respond to the treatment.

The CC response is monitored using pelvic ultrasonography starting on menstrual cycle day 12.

The follicle should develop to a diameter of 23-24 mm before a spontaneous LH surge occurs.

BBT can be used to observe the thermogenic shift induced by the early secretion of progesterone.

The only disadvantage with BBT is that in many instances, the shift does not occur in a clear way, and the patient misses the time of ovulation.

While BBT is an inexpensive way to monitor ovulation, it is often impractical.

Urinary monitoring of the LH surge (eg, with an LH Predictor Kit) can be a substitute for BBT.

The patient should start monitoring the urinary LH secretion daily starting on menstrual cycle day 12.

Ovulation usually occurs within the 32-40 hours after the indicative color change.

Serum LH determination is more precise, especially when performed in combination with pelvic ultrasonography.

Because of the antiestrogenic effect, CC may thicken the cervical mucus, creating an iatrogenic cervical factor that can be responsible for the lack of pregnancy in a patient who has otherwise ovulated.

Other adverse effects associated with CC are hot flashes, scotomas, dryness of the vagina, headache, and ovarian hyperstimulation, which, although rare, has been reported in patients who are sensitive to CC.

The principal indications for CC use are oligomenorrhea, especially PCOS, and for patients with slight menstrual irregularities.

The use of CC is contraindicated in cases of ovarian cyst, pregnancy, and liver disease.

Its use is controversial in patients with a history of breast cancer.

Tamoxifen

Tamoxifen is another SERM, similar to clomiphene that is typically used in the treatment of breast cancer.

Tamoxifen can also be used for ovulation induction.

But, unlike clomiphene, it does not have an anti-estrogenic effect on the uterus.

However, some studies indicate there may be an increased risk for miscarriage with tamoxifen use.

The typical dose is 20 mg daily for 5 days in the early follicular phase, similar to clomiphene.

Success rates with its use are similar to those of clomiphene.

Aromatase Inhibitors

Aromatase inhibitors inhibit the action of the enzyme aromatase, which converts androgens into estrogens by a process called aromatization.

As a result, estrogen levels are dramatically reduced, releasing the hypothalamic-pituitary axis from its negative feedback.

Aromatase inhibitors are FDA approved for treatment of postmenopausal breast cancer, but not for ovulation induction.

When used in the early follicular phase, letrozole inhibits estrogen synthesis, thereby causing enhanced GnRH pulsatility and consequent FSH and inhibin stimulation.

This results in normal or enhanced follicular recruitment without the risk of multiple ovulation and ovarian hyperstimulation.

Letrozole has a very short half-life (45 hours) and, therefore, is quickly cleared from the body.

For this reason, it is less likely to adversely affect the endometrium and cervical mucus.

In a recent meta-analysis, letrozole was found to be as effective as other methods of ovulation induction.

The usual dose for letrozole ovulation induction is 2.5 mg on cycle days 3-7, however, the optimal dosage and length of administration is under investigation.

Aromatase inhibitors are generally well tolerated.

The main side effects are hot flushes, gastrointestinal events (nausea and vomiting), headache, back pain, and leg cramps.

These adverse effects were reported in older women with advanced breast cancer who were given the drugs on a daily basis over several months.

In younger women taking them at lower doses for a short period of time, fewer adverse effects are noted.

The use of aromatase inhibitors for ovulation induction in premenopausal women is controversial due to the possibility of fetal toxicity and fetal malformations.

Furthermore, based on the half-life, administration in the early follicular phase should result in clearance of the aromatase inhibitors before implantation takes place.

Dopamine Agonists

Dopamine agonists are agents that can be used for restoration of ovulation in women with galactorrhea or hyperprolactinemia.

Two agents are available for use, bromocriptine and cabergoline.

Cabergoline is more selective, as it binds specifically to dopamine 2 receptors on the lactotrope cells, and thus has fewer side effects.

Dopamine agonists function like dopamine; they suppress prolactin synthesis and release from the pituitary.

By normalizing the prolactin level, the hypothalamic-pituitary-ovarian axis can return to normal function.

The two drugs are administered slightly differently, although a key component of the use of both is to start at a low dose and titrate up slowly.

Bromocriptine is given at an initial dose of 1.25 mg at bedtime for one week, then increased to twice daily for a month.

A prolactin level can be checked at that time, and if not within normal range, the dose can be increased to 2.5 mg, and then 5 mg if needed.

Cabergoline is given at a dose of 0.25 mg twice a week.

This is increased to 0.5 mg, and then 1.0 mg, twice a week, if after a month at each dose the prolactin level is not yet in normal range.

A response to treatment can be seen by a drop in the serum prolactin level 2-3 weeks after the initiation of therapy.

Normalization of serum prolactin levels should be accompanied by normal menstrual cycles.

Dopamine agonists are successful for treating anovulation; 80% of women will ovulate after correction of hyperprolactinemia, with cumulative pregnancy rates of 70-80%.

Adverse effects for both drugs include dizziness, nausea, and hypotension.

Cabergoline is better tolerated, as it is the more selective of the two drugs.

Both can be administered vaginally to improve tolerability.

Gonadotropins

Human menopausal gonadotropin (hMG) contains 75 U of FSH and 75 U of LH per mL, although the concentration may vary among batches.

In the 1980s, a pure form of FSH became available; urofollitropin contains 75 U of FSH.

The new generations of available gonadotropins are produced by genetically engineered mammalian cells, in which the gene coding for the alpha and beta FSH subunits has been inserted.

Recombinant LH may be added to recombinant FSH protocols as an alternative, particularly useful in patients with hypothalamic amenorrhea.

The administration of hMG and its derivatives should be under the direct supervision of a reproductive endocrinologist.

An ultrasonography unit and an endocrine laboratory capable of performing daily determinations of E_2, FSH, and LH are necessary.

Multiple adverse effects and complications may occur during the use of the gonadotropins, including

– Multiple pregnancy (24-33%),

– Ectopic pregnancy (5-8%),

– Miscarriages (15-21%),

– Ovarian torsion and rupture, and

– Ovarian hyperstimulation syndrome (OHSS).

The increase of ovarian cancer associated with infertility might be due to the use of fertility drugs.

hMG and its derivatives are indicated for ovulation induction in patients with primary amenorrhea due to hypopituitarism and in patients with secondary amenorrhea who did not respond to CC ovulation induction.

For the past 20 years, hMG and its derivatives have been the first choice for controlled ovarian hyperstimulation in assisted reproductive technologies.

Human Chorionic Gonadotropins (hCG)

hCG is available in two preparations, similar to the gonadotropins: purified urinary hCG and recombinant hCG.

hCG is used for triggering final follicular maturation and/or ovulation.

It can provide this function because it is very similar in structure to LH.

Both hormones contain the same alpha subunit; however, the beta subunit is also very similar, so hCG can bind to and activate the LH receptor.

When used to trigger ovulation, a dose of 5,000-10,000 IU of urinary hCG is typically given by intramuscular or subcutaneous injection.

Other doses have also been used.

The dose of recombinant hCG that is used is 250 mcg, given by subcutaneous injection, which is roughly equivalent to 6,000 IU of hCG.

There is no difference in pregnancy outcomes between urinary and recombinant forms.

Lower doses have been suggested as a means for reducing the risk of OHSS.

However, the efficacy of this approach has not been proven in randomized controlled trials.

When hCG is used as an ovulation trigger, ultrasound is used to monitor follicle size and time administration of hCG.

Ovulation will occur 36-44 hours following the injection.

Gonadotropin Releasing Hormone

Synthetic GnRH has a chemical composition similar to native GnRH and is indicated for patients with hypothalamic dysfunction, especially those who do not respond to CC.

This drug is administered in a pulsatile fashion every 60-120 minutes, intravenously or subcutaneously using a delivery pump.

The starting dose is 5 mcg per pulse intravenously or 5-25 mcg subcutaneously.

The administration on GnRH should be extended throughout the luteal phase, or this should be supplemented with the administration of exogenous hCG.

Monitoring folliculogenesis is simpler than using hMG.

Pelvic ultrasonography can be used once a week until the dominant follicle is detected; once this occurs, ultrasonography can be used more frequently until ovulation occurs.

Determination of serum E_2 and LH levels can also be performed.

Gonadotropin Releasing Hormone Antagonists

Similar to the GnRH agonists, GnRH antagonists were developed by modification of the native GnRH protein.

Two products are marketed for use in US: cetrorelix and ganirelix.

Both function to antagonize GnRH by binding and blocking the GnRH receptor from signaling.

They are used in controlled ovarian stimulation IVF cycles to prevent a premature LH surge.

Both compounds are formulated as a 0.25 mg subcutaneous injection that is given daily to suppress the LH surge.

Treatment is typically started when the lead follicle reaches a diameter of 14 mm, or when estradiol levels reach 400 pg/mL.

The antagonist is then continued daily until ovulation trigger.

Cetrorelix can also be given as a single dose of 3 mg subcutaneously on day 8 or 9 of stimulation; this may need to be repeated if stimulation continues for more than 3 additional days.

Routine monitoring of controlled ovarian stimulation with serial estradiol levels and ultrasounds is performed; one can anticipate a blunting of the estradiol response as a result of starting antagonist therapy.

Primary Amenorrhea

hMG is the treatment of choice for patients with hypopituitarism.

The risk of OHSS and multiple pregnancy is heightened; therefore, hMG should be started at the minimal dose (75 IU SC qd for 7 d).

On the seventh day, E_2 measurement and ultrasonography are performed.

If the E_2 is below 100 pc/mL and the sonogram shows small follicular development, hMG is increased to 150 IU/d for an additional 5 days.

However, if the E_2 is greater than 100 pc/mL and the follicles are 10 mm in diameter, hMG should be continued at the same dose.

Once the follicular diameter reaches 18 mm and the E_2 level is below 2000 pc/mL, ovulation is triggered by the administration of hCG (10,000 IU IM).

The ideal response is one in which only 2-3 follicles develop.

If the response is exaggerated, with more than 5 sizable follicles (18 mm in diameter), and the E_2 level is greater than 2500 pc/mL, cancelling the ovulation is better to avoid the risk of OHSS and a high order of multiple pregnancy.

In current practice, an alternative for patients with more than 5 sizable follicles is to convert the treatment to IVF.

Secondary Amenorrhea

Once the diagnosis is established and any other endocrinopathy has been excluded, the ovulation induction agent of choice depends on a functioning hypothalamic-pituitary-ovarian axis.

In patients with low gonadotropins and low estrogen, the treatment of choice is hMG, and the protocol is similar to that for patients with primary amenorrhea.

If the E_2 and FSH levels are in the normal range, CC is the drug of choice, as previously described.

PCOS is the most frequent indication for ovulation induction.

CC is the drug of choice.

Restrict the treatment to 4 ovulatory cycles because 85% of patients conceive by the fourth ovulatory cycle.

If pregnancy is not achieved, further evaluation is required to exclude other factors that may be associated with infertility and may interfere with the success of CC therapy.

If ovulation does not occur with the 50-mg dose, the CC dose must be increased in subsequent cycles to maximum 150 mg for 5 days.

Most recommend dosing CC on cycle days 3-7 to improve response and ovulation around cycle day 14.

Lack of Ovulation

Patients with anovulation who did not ovulate after several cycles of CC at different doses of treatment are deemed clomiphene resistant.

This situation can be related to the presence of other endocrine disorders such as hyperprolactinemia, congenital adrenal hyperplasia, adrenal tumors, Cushing syndrome, thyroid dysfunction, and extreme obesity.

Therefore, this problem must be corrected first or concomitantly to obtain an ovulatory response.

A subgroup of PCOS patients has hyperinsulinism, hyperandrogenism associated with acanthosis nigricans, and resistance to CC; this group is amenable to metformin treatment.

Metformin improves insulin sensitivity and decreases hepatic gluconeogenesis and, therefore, reduces hyperinsulinism, basal and stimulated LH levels, and free testosterone concentration.

Adverse effects of metformin include GI intolerance, nausea, vomiting, and abdominal cramps.

Weight loss has also been observed, therefore, patients must build up tolerance.

Pure FSH treatment for ovulation induction is another alternative for patients with PCOS who are clomiphene resistant.

Lack of Pregnancy

Lack of pregnancy can be related to disruption of the cervical mucus, inadequate follicular development, presence of luteinized unruptured follicle syndrome, progesterone deficiency, and premature administration of hCG to trigger ovulation.

The quality of the cervical mucus can be improved with the administration of a small dose of estrogens, or the problem can be bypassed by intrauterine insemination (IUI).

If the follicle is smaller than 23-24 mm at the time of ovulation, a better size can be obtained by starting the CC therapy on cycle day 2.

Luteinized unruptured follicle syndrome can be prevented by the administration of hCG (10,000 IU IM) once the follicle reaches 23-24 mm in diameter.

Progesterone deficiency can be corrected by the administration of progesterone during the luteal phase, starting 48 hours after ovulation.

Ovulation usually occur 5 days after the last dose of CC, however, ovulation may occur between day 1 and day 14 after the last tablet of CC is administered; thus, pelvic ultrasonography has become an important tool for monitoring ovulation induction.

Weight reduction should be part of the treatment because it helps the patient's response to ovulation induction.

OVARIAN STIMULATION FOR IVF

Controlled ovarian hyperstimulation (COH) is frequently used with IVF cycles, as it does improve pregnancy rates.

Exact protocols vary by clinic, but involve the use of injectable gonadotropins.

The use of an oral contraceptive prior to treatment may minimize cycle cancellation and allow for greater control of cycle management.

A commonly-used stimulation protocol uses a combination of GnRH agonists and gonadotropins.

Natural cycle IVF (using no medications) and minimal stimulation protocols (using oral ovulation-induction agents) are other possibilities, but the yield of oocytes and embryos, and thus pregnancy rates, are significantly lower.

These alternatives are useful for avoiding OHSS and decreasing the chances of a multiple pregnancy.

The aim of all stimulation protocols is to induce the development of a cohort of equidominant follicles in both ovaries.

The success rate in any one IVF cycle has been clearly shown to be increased form 4.2% in a natural cycle to 17% in a stimulated cycle where more than one embryo is transferred.

An increased number of eggs at the time of oocyte retrieval is directly linked to a significant improvement in pregnancy rates.

Stimulation regimens are designed with the following aims:

– To prevent premature luteinization.

– To prevent spontaneous ovulation.

– To improve endometrial response.

– To allow greater flexibility for ambulatory patient management, with reduced cycle monitoring, and the giving of injections at home.

Modifications to stimulation protocols are continually being reviewed:

– The protocol needs to be tailored to each individual patient in order to maximize the prospect of success whilst minimizing complications.

– Emphasis is given to a team approach in the making of decisions regarding stimulation; usually the patient's clinician, liaising with the nurse practitioner directly involved with the patient's care, and the embryologist, if necessary in consultation with a specialist endocrinologist, will meet to decide the most appropriate protocol.

– Varied protocols of COH have been developed based on the use of the agents described; ongoing modifications will occur depending on the patient's response, newer agents and the results of treatment.

The use of GnRH agonists and antagonists with gonadotropins has resulted in greater ease of planning the supervoulation stimulation than was possible with the earlier use of CC with gonadotropin.

That regimen had to be monitored carefully in order to predict and prevent the occurrence of an endogenous prevoulatory LH surge.

In the absence of GnRH controlled cycles there is a cancellation rate of 15% because oocyte retrieval has to be performed 26 hours after the detection of the endogenous surge and this often meant that oocyte collections were performed at night and at weekends.

When GnRH agonists or antagonists are used, the oocyte retrieval can be precisely timed to occur 34 hours after the administration of hCG.

hCG acts as a surrogate for the normal mid-cycle LH surge, and causes resumption of meiosis within the oocytes and their preparation for fertilization.

Furthermore, there is good evidence that the oocytes do not become overmature within follicles that are considered to be ready for collection and so the administration of hCG can be delayed to avoid oocyte collection at weekends.

Success rates appear to be better when GnRH agonists are used and the rates of miscarriage, especially in PCOS, appear to be reduced.

Most stimulation regimens commence the day after menses has started (i.e., day 2) for practical reasons.

A day 1 start is acceptable but often not practical as most clinics like to communicate with their patients when they are about to start treatment.

Alternatively, the combined oral contraceptive pill can be used to program the cycle.

Pituitary desensitization "downregulatin" has occurred when the serum concentration of LH is <5 IU/L and that of estradiol <50 pg/mL (progesterone, if measured, should be <3 mmol/L).

hCG or recombinant LH is given to trigger oocyte maturation when the largest follicle reaches at least 18 mm in diameter and there are at least two others >17 mm; oocyte collection is performed 35 hours later; ET occurs approximately 48 hours after oocyte collection.

Luteal support commences the day of ET and is usually given as progesterone suppositories or IM injections and continued until the day of the pregnancy test.

Some continue luteal support up to 12 weeks' gestation, although this is unnecessary if progesterone pessaries have been used.

Long Protocol

A disadvantage of the use of GnRH agonists is the 2 weeks or more lead-in to the therapy during which pituitary desensitization "down-regulation" is achieved before stimulation with gonadotropins can be commenced.

Some clinics prefer to commence agonist therapy on day 21 of the cycle and suggest that desensitization occurs more rapidly than if it is commenced during menstruation - usually day 2.

A day 21 start, however, carries the risk of "rescuing" a corpus luteum with resultant functional cyst formation; a day 2 start virtually guarantees that the patient is not pregnant.

Combined oral contraceptive pill can be administered for between 2 and 3 weeks commencing on day 1 of the menstrual cycle.

This regimen allows scheduling of cycles in a busy clinic and also the use of the contraceptive pill minimizes the occurrence of ovarian cysts resulting from the GnRH agonist "flare".

The disadvantage, of course, is further prolongation of the treatment cycle.

The GnRH agonists can be administered intranasally, subcutaneously, or intramuscularly.

Short and Ultrashort Protocols

The shorter acting preparations can be used to induce a flare response, being commenced on day 1 of the cycle, with gonadotropin stimulation starting the following day.

The agonist is then either continued through to the day of hCG "short protocol" or given for 3 days only "ultrashort protocol".

The flare response can be utilized in those patients who have had a poor response in the past in order to try to maximize the response to stimulation - this it does to varying degrees.

It is, in fact, difficult to predict an individual's response to stimulation: young women and those with PCOS tend to respond well, while older patients and those with elevated baseline serum concentrations of FSH (>10 IU/L on most assays) respond less well.

CC and GnRH stimulation tests have been employed to improve the predictability of response but do not tend to be highly sensitive.

An assessment of ovarian volume, antral follicle count and anti-Müllerian hormone (AMH) concentration have become popular in assessing ovarian reserve.

Antagonist Protocol

The advent of the third-generation GnRH antagonist enables us to dispense with pituitary densitization and commence ovarian stimulation on day 2, with the daily administration of an antagonist on day 6 of stimulation or once the leading follicle(s) has reached a diameter of 14 mm (usually day 6 or 7); however, it appears that success rates are better when commenced on day 6 rather than using a flexible protocol.

GnRH antagonists act immediately to inhibit pituitary secretion of FSH and LH without the flare effect of antagonists or the need for 10 days' desensitization; an endogenous LH surge can be prevented, thereby allowing oocyte retrieval at the desired time.

GnRH antagonist cycles are certainly much shorter and more convenient for patients than the "long protocol" and many clinics are now increasingly using them.

Oocyte maturation prior to collection may be initiated with a single shot of a GnRH agonist rather than hCG - a strategy that was proposed to reduce the risk of OHSS because of the shorter half-life of the agonist compared with hCG; however pregnancy rates are lower and so the conventional use of hCG is recommended.

The use of GnRH antagonists may also reduce the total requirement for gonadotropins and obviate any need for luteal support.

GnRH antagonist cycles may be preferred because of their short duration and minimal side effects (for example, avoidance of symptoms of estrogen deficiency during pituitary desensitization).

1. Clomiphene citrate plus gonadotropins (hMG or FSH)

```
|menses (day 1)                                          oocyte collection ▫
    |clomiphene 100 mg per day
     day 2 for 5 days
        |gonadotropin stimulation from day 4 to day of hCG|
                                                         hCG ▫
```

2. Long GnRH agonist protocols

a. Luteal phase start (i.e., 7 days after presumed day of ovulation)

```
|ovulation              |menses                  oocyte collection ▫
        |GnRH agonist day 21   |drop dose, continue to
                                day of hCG
                               |gonadotropins to day of hCG|
                                                         hCG ▫
```

b. Follicular phase start

```
|menses                                          oocyte collection ▫
    |GnRH agonist starts day 2 until |drop dose, continue to
     "downregulation,"                day of hCG
     usually 14 days
                                     |gonadotropins to day of hCG|
                                                         hCG ▫
```

3. Short GnRH agonist protocol

```
|menses (day 1)                                  oocyte collection ▫
    |GnRH agonist starts day 2 to day of hCG           |
    |gonadotropin stimulation from day 3 to day of hCG |
                                                         hCG ▫
```

4. Ultra-short GnRH agonist protocol

```
|menses (day 1)                                  oocyte collection ▫
    |GnRH agonist from
     day 2 for 3 days
        |gonadotropin stimulation from day 3 to day of hCG|
                                                         hCG ▫
```

5. GnRH antagonist protocol (a GnRH agonist can be given instead of hCG)

```
|menses (day 1)                                  oocyte collection ▫
    |gonadotropin stimulation from day 2 to day of hCG|
        daily injection of antagonist when leading follicle 14 mm ▫
                                                         hCG ▫
```

Ovarian Stimulation Protocols for IVF

Gonadotropin Therapy for IVF

Gonadotropin therapy for the stimulation of superovulation can be with either hMG, which contains urinary-derived FSH and LH in differing proportions depending on the preparation, or with urinary-derived FSH alone, which is available for administration subcutaneously because of its higher purity.

The original sources of gonadotropins for therapeutic use were post-mortem pituitary extracts and the urine of postmenopausal women.

The former source was withdrawn because of cases of Creutzfeldt-Jakob disease, which occurred predominantly in Australia and Europe.

The extraction and purification of postmenopausal urine were pioneered in Italy in the late 1940s to result in the production of hMG.

Twenty to thirty liters of postmenopausal urine were required to provide sufficient gonaodtropin for one cycle of hMG.

Through the 1960s the extraction process to remove non-specific co-purified proteins became more sophisticated, such that activity was increased 10 fold over the early preparations.

Greater purity produced fewer hypersensitivity reactions and less discomfort from the smaller volume of the injection.

Clinical trials comparing uFSH (urofollitropin) and highly purified FSH demonstrated equivalent ovulation and pregnancy rates.

Reduced hypersensitivity was reported, such that the subcutaneous route could be adopted for administration.

However, the problems of supply, collection, transport, storage, and processing of an ever increasing requirement of urine remained and the pharmaceutical companies have now utilized the technology of genetic engineering to produce biosynthetic preparations.

The genes for the alfa and beta subunits of FSH were incorporated into vectors which were then introduced into cells from a Chinese hamster ovary cell line; this process has resulted in an unlimited supply of highly stable therapeutic preparations with a high specific activity.

The advent of the recombinant gonadotropins has broadened the scope of therapeutic agents and resulted in a potentially unlimited supply.

To date there are two recombinant FSH preparations: follitropin alfa (Gonal-F, Serono) and follitropin beta (Puregon, Organon).

In discussing the benefits of a gonadotropin preparation one has to consider clinical efficacy, side effects and cost-effectiveness.

Clinical efficacy includes the ability to stimulate folliculogenesis, the production of mature oocytes, appropriate steroidogenesis for endometrial development and, in the context of IVF, sufficient quality pre-embryos and, ultimately, good rates of pregnancy.

Monitoring the Treatment Cycle

The monitoring of follicular response to superovulation requires a combination of parameters.

Specifically, there needs to be vaginal ultrasound assessment of follicular size and number, and measurements of plasma estradiol, LH and progesterone levels need to be ascertained

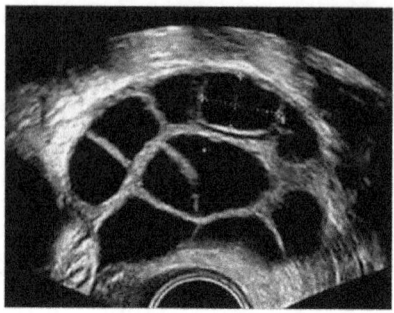

Ovarian Stimulation for IVF

The patient's history and current treatment are scrutinized together with the current results.

Decisions concerning changes in management, cycle cancellation alteration in drug dosage, timing of hCG and oocyte recovery are conveyed promptly to the patient.

<u>Criteria for Cycle Cancellatio</u>

−Abnormal findings seen on ultrasound scan.

−Falling estradiol levels despite increased stimulation.

−Estradiol >6000 pg/mL; if hyperstimulation occurs, consider continuing GnRH agonist down regulation until the ovaries are quiescent.

OVARIAN HYPERSTIMULATION SYNDROME

Ovarian hyperstimulation syndrome (OHSS) is an iatrogenic condition that occurs in patients undergoing ovulation induction with hMG or controlled ovarian hyperstimulation for IVF.

The pathophysiology is not well understood, but a massive extravascular accumulation of fluid occurs that is associated with depletion of intravascular volume responsible for dehydration, hemoconcentration, and electrolyte imbalance (hyponatremia, hyperkalemia).

Risk factors of OHSS

−Young women (<35 years).

−PCOS.

−Large number of follicles with a high portion of small and intermediate follicles.

−High and rapid rise of serum estradiol.

−PCOS pattern for response to GnRH before hMG.

−Conception cycles, particularly multiple pregnancies.

−OHSS in a previous cycle.

−GnRH agonist use.

−Luteal phase supplementation with hCG.

−Multiple pregnancy.

Classification of OHSS

Mild OHSS

Ovarian enlargement (up to 5-12 cm in diameter), minimal ascites, and weight gain of less than 10 lb.

Moderate OHSS

Ovarian enlargement (5-12 cm in diameter), moderate ascites, nausea, vomiting, abdominal discomfort, and weight gain greater than 10 lb.

Severe OHSS

Easily palpable ovaries, severe ascites, nausea, vomiting, diarrhea, shortness of breath, hydrothorax, peripheral edema, oliguria, hemoconcentration (eg, hematocrit level >48% and hemoglobin level >16 g), and creatinine level greater than 1.6 mg/dL.

Renal failure and thrombosis can occur if the patient is not treated correctly.

Prediction of OHSS

The majority of cases can be predicted by the combined use of ultrasound and endocrine monitoring.

In case where estradiol was >6000 pg/mL, there is a greater chance of developing severe OHSS.

A decrease in the fraction of mature follicles and an increase in the fraction of the very small follicles (>15) were associated with an increased risk of OHSS.

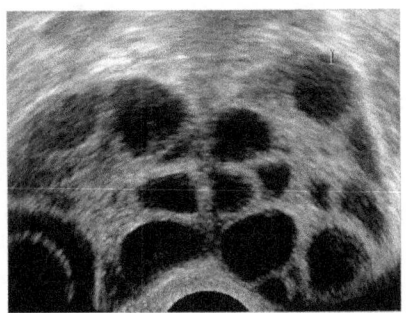

Ovarian Hyperstimulation Syndrome (OHSS)

Prevention of OHSS

- Withholding hCG and cancellation of the IVF cycle.

- Reducing the dose of hCG to 5000 IU.

- Delaying hCG for several days (coasting).

- GnRH agonists to trigger ovulation.

- GnRH antagonist protocol.

- Progesterone for luteal phase support.

- Cryopreservation of embryos.

- In vitro maturation (IVM).

- Intravenous albumin administration at the time of oocyte collection.

- Insulin-sensitizing agents (metformin).

- Dopamine agonist (cabergoline) administration.

Treatment of OHSS

OHSS is self-limited, and the symptoms subside within 2-6 weeks.

Patients with mild and moderate OHSS are treated at home with bedrest and strict control of fluid intake and output.

If a weight gain greater than 2 lb occurs, the patient should be evaluated to determine if hospitalization is required.

Patients with severe OHSS are often hospitalized and confined to bed, with strict control of fluid intake and output.

Intravenous fluids (ie, isotonic sodium chloride solution) must be administered until hemodilution is achieved.

If the urinary output remains low, albumin 25% (50 mL/h IV for 4 h) has been effective in promoting diuresis.

Transvaginal or abdominal paracentesis should be performed if the patient becomes uncomfortable.

Because of the risk of thrombosis, heparin (5000 U SC q12h) is recommended.

Some have had success treating severe OHSS on an outpatient basis by performing aggressive transvaginal paracentesis with good outcomes.

REFERENCES

- Al-Azemi M, Killick S, Duffy S, et al. Multi-marker assessment of ovarian reserve predicts oocyte yield after ovulation induction. Hum Reprod. 2011; 26: 414-22.

- Al-Inany H, Abou-Setta A, Aboulghar M. GnRH antagonists for ART. Cochrane Database Syst Rev. 2006; 3: CD001750.

- American Society for Reproductive Medicine. Use of clomiphene citrate in women. ASRM Committee Opinion. Fertil Steril. 2006; 86: S187-93.

- American Society for Reproductive Medicine. Use of exogenous gonadotropins in anovulatory women. ASRM Technical Bulletin. Fertil Steril. 2008; 90: S7-12.

- American Society for Reproductive Medicine. Gonadotropin preparations: past, present, and future perspectives. ASRM Educational Bulletin. Fertil Steril. 2008; 90: S13-20.

- American Society for Reproductive Medicine. Current Evaluation of amenorrhea. ASRM Practice Committee. Fertil Steril. 2008; 90: S219-25.

- Badawy A, Mosbah A, Tharwat A, et al. Extended letrozole therapy for ovulation induction in clomiphene-resistant women with polycystic ovary syndrome: a novel protocol. Fertil Steril. 2009; 92: 236-9.

- Balen A, St James. Assisted conception. In: Adam H Balen, editor. Infertility in practice, 3rd edition. Informa Healthcare; 2008.

- Bedaiwy M, Mousa N, Esfandiari N, et al. Follicular phase dynamics with combined aromatase inhibitor and follicle stimulating hormone treatment. J Clin Endocrinol Metab. 2007; 92: 825-33.

- Bellver J, Munoz E, Ballesteros A, et al. Intravenous albumin does not prevent moderate-severe OHSS in high-risk IVF patients: A randomized controlled study. Hum Reprod. 2003; 18: 2283-8.

References

- Berin I, Stein DE, Keltz M. A comparison of gonadotropin-releasing hormone (GnRH) antagonist and GnRH agonist flare protocols for poor responders undergoing in vitro fertilization. Fertil Steril. 2010; 93: 360-3.

- Broekmans F, Kwee J, Hendriks D, et al. A systematic review of tests predicting ovarian reserve and IVF outcome. Hum Reprod Update. 2006; 12: 685-718.

- Caburet S, Arboleda V, Llano E, et al. Mutant Cohesin in Premature Ovarian Failure. N Engl J Med. 2014; 370: 943-9.

- Carizza C, Abdelmassih V, Abdelmassih S, et al. Cabergoline reduces the early onset of OHSS: A prospective randomized study. RBM Online. 2008; 17: 751-5.

- Casper R, Mitwally M. Review: aromatase inhibitors for ovulation induction. J Clin Endocrinol Metab. 2006; 91: 760-71.

- Chung K. Gross Anatomy. 4th ed. Philadelphia: Lippincott Williams & Wilkins; 2000.

- Costello M, Chapman M, Conway U. A systematic review and meta-analysis of randomized controlled trials on metformin co-administration during gonadotropin ovulation induction or IVF in women with PCOS. Hum Reprod. 2006; 21: 1387-99.

- Coviello A, Legro R, Dunaif A. Adolescent girls with polycystic ovary syndrome have an increased risk of the metabolic syndrome associated with increasing androgen levels independent of obesity and insulin resistance. J Clin Endocrinol Metab. 2006; 92: 492-7.

- Daya S. GnRH agonist protocols for pituitary desensitization in IVF and GIFT cycles. Cochrane Database of Systematic Reviews 2000; 1: CD001299.

- Daya S. Updated meta-analysis of recombinant follicle-stimulating hormone (FSH) versus urinary FSH for ovarian stimulation in assisted reproduction. Fertil Steril. 2002; 77: 711-4.

- Delvigne A, Rozenberg S. Epidemiology and prevention of OHSS: A review. Hum Reprod Update. 2002; 8: 559-77.

- Dickey R, Holtkamp D. Development, pharmacology, and clinical experience with clomiphene citrate. Hum Reprod Update. 1996; 2: 483-506.

- Donckers J, Evers J, Land J. The long-term outcome of 946 consecutive couples visiting a fertility clinic in 2001-2003. Fertil Steril. 2011; 96: 160-4.

- Dovey S, Sneeringer R, Penzias A. Clomiphene citrate and intrauterine insemination: analysis of more than 4100 cycles. Fertil Steril. 2008; 90: 2281-6.

- Drake R, Vogl A, Mitchell A. Gray's Anatomy for Student's. 2nd ed. Philadelphia: Churchill Livingstone Elsevier; 2010.

- Eftekhari N, Mohammadalizadeh S. Pregnancy rate following bromocriptine treatment in infertile women with galactorrhea. Gynecol Endocrinol. 2009; 25: 122-4.

- Engmann L, DiLuigi A, Schmidt D, et al. The use of gonadotropin-releasing hormone (GnRH) agonist to induce oocyte maturation after cotreatment with GnRH antagonist in high-risk patients undergoing in vitro fertilization prevents the risk of ovarian hyperstimulation syndrome: a prospective randomized controlled study. Fertil Steril. 2008; 89: 84-91.

- European Orgalutran Study Group, Borm G, Mannaerts B. Treatment with the GnRH antagonist ganirelix in women undergoing COH with recombinant FSH is effective, safe and convenient: results of controlled, randomized, multicenter trial. Hum Reprod. 2000; 15: 1490-8.

- Ferraretti A, Gianaroli L, Magli MC, et al. Female poor responders. Mol Cell Endocrinol. 2000; 161: 59-66.

- Fisch J, Keskintepe L, Sher G. GnRH agonist/antagonist conversion with estrogen priming in low responders with prior IVF failure. Fertil Steril. 2008; 89: 342-7.

References

- Forman R, Gill S, Moretti M, et al. Fetal safety of letrozole and clomiphene citrate for ovulation induction. J Obstet Gynaecol Can. 2007; 29: 668-71.

- Freizinger M, Franko D, Dacey M, et al. The prevalence of eating disorders in infertile women. Fertil. Steril. 2008; 93: 72-8.

- Gray H. Anatomy, Descriptive and Surgical. The Unabridged Gray's Anatomy. Philadelphia: Running Press; 1999.

- Heijnen E, Eijkemans M, Hughes E, et al. A meta-analysis of outcomes of conventional IVF in women with PCOS. Hum Reprod Update. 2006; 12: 13-21.

- Huang H, Lv C, Zhao Y, et al. Mutant ZP1 in Familial Infertility. N Engl J Med. 2014; 370: 1220-6.

- Imani B, Eijkemans M, te Velde E, et al. A nomogram to predict the probability of live birth after clomiphene citrate induction of ovulation in normogonadotropic oligoamenorrheic infertility. Fertil Steril. 2002; 77: 91-7.

- Isik A, Vicdan K. Combined approach as an effective method in the prevention of severe OHSS. EJOGRB. 2001; 97: 208-12.

- Kallio S, Aittomäki K, Piltonen T, et al. Anti-Mullerian hormone as a predictor of follicular reserve in ovarian insufficiency: special emphasis on FSH-resistant ovaries. Hum Reprod. 2012; 27: 854-60.

- Kashyap S, Parker K, Cedars M, et al. Ovarian hyperstimulation syndrome prevention strategies: reducing the human chorionic gonadotropin trigger dose. Semin Reprod Med. 2010; 28: 475-85.

- Katz V, Lentz G, Lobo R, et al. Comprehensive Gynecology. 5th ed. Philadelphia: Mosby Elsevier; 2007.

- Kligman I, Rosenwaks Z. Differentiating clinical profiles: predicting good responders, poor responders, and hyperresponders. Fertil Steril. 2001; 76: 1185-90.

- Knochenhauer E, Key T, Kahsar-Miller M, et al. Prevalence of the polycystic ovary syndrome in unselected black and white women of the southeastern United States: a prospective study. J Clin Endocrinol Metab. 1998; 83: 3078-82.

- Kolodziejczyk B, Duleba A, Spaczynski R, et al. Metformin therapy decreases hyperandrogenism and hyperinsulinemia in women with polycystic ovary syndrome. Fertil Steril. 2000; 73: 1149-54.

- Konig E, Bussen S, Sutterlin M, et al. Prophylactic intravenous hydroxyethyl starch solution prevents moderate-severe ovarian hyperstimulation in IVF patients: a prospective, randomized, double-blind and placebo-controlled study. Hum Reprod. 1998; 13: 2421-4.

- Koning A, Kuchenbecker W, Groen H, et al. Economic consequences of overweight and obesity in infertility: a framework for evaluating the costs and outcomes of fertility care. Hum Reprod Update. 2010; 16: 246-54.

- Kovacs G. IVF: indications, stimulation and clinical Techniques. In: James MCK, Mark L, editors. The subfertility handbook, 1st edition. Cambridge University Press; 1997.

- Laughlin G, Dominguez C, Yen S. Nutritional and endocrine-metabolic aberrations in women with functional hypothalamic amenorrhea. J Clin Endocrinol Metab. 1998; 83: 25-32.

- Legro R, Barnhart H, Schlaff W, et al. Cooperative Multicenter Reproductive Medicine Network. Clomiphene, metformin, or both for infertility in the polycystic ovary syndrome. N Engl J Med. 2007; 356: 551-66.

- Liu J, Aziz R, Dodson W, et al, editors. Précis – Reproductive Endocrinology, 3rd edition. Washington, DC: ACOG; 2007.

- Loh S, Wang J, Matthews C. The influence of BMI, basal FSH and age on the response to gonadotropin stimulation in non-PCOS patients. Hum Reprod. 2002; 17: 1207-11.

References

- Lord J, Flight I, Norman R. Metformin in polycystic ovary syndrome: systematic review and meta-analysis. BMJ. 2003; 327: 951-3.

- Loukas M, Colburn G, Abrahams P, et al. Gray's Anatomy Review. Philadelphia: Churchill Livingstone Elsevier; 2010.

- Lyons C, Wheeler C, Frishman G, et al. Early and late presentation of the ovarian hyperstimulation syndrome: two distinct entities with different risk factors. Hum Reprod. 1994; 9: 792-9.

- Macklon D, Fauser C. Medical approaches to ovarian stimulation for infertility. In: Jerome I, Robert M, eds. Yen & Jaffe's Reproductive Endocrinology, 6th Edition Vol. 28. Philadelphia: Saunders, 2009: 698-708.

- Macklon N, Stouffer R, Giudice L, et al. The science behind 25 years of ovarian stimulation for IVF. Endocr Rev. 2006; 27: 170-207.

- Marcus M, Loucks T, Berga S. Psychological correlates of functional hypothalamic amenorrhea. Fertil Steril. 2001; 76: 310-6.

- Mulders A, Laven J, Eijkemans M, et al. Patient predictors for outcome of gonadotrophin ovulation induction in women with normogonadotrophic anovulatory infertility: a meta-analysis. Hum Reprod Update. 2003; 9: 429-49.

- Mulders A, Laven J, Imani B, et al. IVF outcome in anovulatory infertility (WHO group 2) including PCOS-following previous unsuccessful ovulation induction. RBM Online. 2003; 7: 50-8.

- Neill J. Knobil and Neill's Physiology of Reproduction. 3rd ed. St. Louis, MO: Elsevier; 2006.

- Ovalle W, Nahirney P. Netter's Eseential Histology. Philadelphia: Sauders Elsevier; 2007.

- Pandian Z, Gibreel A, Bhattacharya S. In vitro fertilisation for unexplained subfertility. Cochrane Database Syst Rev. 2015; 11: CD003357.

References

- Pasquali R, Gambineri A, Pagotto U. The impact of obesity on reproduction in women with PCOS. BJOG. 2006; 113: 1148-59.

- Pierpoint T, McKeigue P, Isaacs A, et al. Mortality of Women with Polycystic Ovary Syndrome at Long-term Follow-up. J Clin Epidemiol. 1998; 51: 581-6.

- Practice Committee of American Society for Reproductive Medicine in collaboration with Society for Reproductive Endocrinology and Infertility. Optimizing natural fertility. Fertil Steril. 2008; 90: S1-6.

- Practice Committee of the American Society for Reproductive Medicine. Optimal evaluation of the infertile female. Fertil Steril. 2006; 86: S264-7.

- Ragni G, Vegetti W, Riccaboni A, et al. Comparison of GnRH agonists and antagonists in ART cycles of patients at high risk of OHSS. Hum Reprod. 2005; 20: 2421-5.

- Reindollar R, Regan M, Neumann P, et al. A randomized clinical trial to evaluate optimal treatment for unexplained infertility: the fast track and standard treatment (FASTT) trial. Fertil Steril. 2010; 94: 888-99.

- Revel A, Casper R. The use of LH-RH agonist to induce ovulation. In: Devroey P, editor. Infertility and Reproductive Medicine Clinics of North America. Philadelphia: WB Saunders; 2001: 105-18.

- Rizk B, Aboulghar M. Classification, pathophysiology and management of OHSS. In: Brinsden PR, editor. A Textbook of IVF and Assisted Reproduction, 2nd edition. Carnforth: Parthenon Publishing; 1999: 131-55.

- Rizk B, Nawar M. OHSS. In: Serhal P, Overton C, editors. Good Clinical Practice in Assisted Reproduction, 1st edition. Cambridge University Press; 2004: 146-66.

- Rotterdam ESHRE/ASRM-Sponsored PCOS Consensus Workshop Group. Revised 2003 consensus on diagnostic criteria and long-term health risks related to polycystic ovary syndrome. Fertil Steril. 2004; 81: 19-25.

References

– Sadler T. Langman's Medical Embryology. 11th ed. Baltimore, Maryland: Lippincott Williams & Wilkins; 2010.

– Seow k, Juan C, Hwang I, et al. Laparoscopic surgery in PCOS: reproductive and metabolic effects. Semin Reprod Med. 2008; 26: 101-11.

– Serhal P, Overton C. Ovarian hyperstimulation syndrome. In: Rizk B, Nawar MG, editors. Good Clinical Practice in Assisted Reproduction, 1st edition. Cambridge University Press; 2004.

– Shavit T, Shalom-Paz E, Samara N, et al. Comparison between stimulation with highly purified hMG or recombinant FSH in patients undergoing IVF with GnRH antagonist protocol. Gynecol Endocrinol. 2016; 3:1-5.

– Smith L, Hacker M, Alper M. Patients with severe ovarian hyperstimulation syndrome can be managed safely with aggressive outpatient transvaginal paracentesis. Fertil Steril. 2009; 92: 1953-9.

– Speroff L, Fritz M, eds. Clinical Gynecologic Endocrinology and Infertility, 7th edition. Philadelphia: Lippincot, Williams & Wilkins, 2005.

– Standring S. Gray's Anatomy. 40th ed. Edinburgh: Elsevier Churchill Livingstone; 2008.

– Sun W, Stegmann B, Henne M, et al. A new approach to ovarian reserve testing. Fertil Steril. 2008; 90: 2196-202.

– Tannus S, Burke Y, Kol S. Treatment strategies for the infertile polycystic ovary syndrome patient. Womens Health (Lond Engl). 2015; 11: 901-12.

– Tarlatzis B, Zepiridis L, Grimbizis G, et al. Clinical management of low ovarian response to stimulation for IVF: a systematic review. Hum Reprod Update. 2003; 9: 61-76.

– Textbook of ARTs: Laboratory and clinical perspectives, 3rd edition. In: Gardner DK, Weissman A, Howles CM, Shoham Z, editors. 2009.

References

- Thessaloniki ESHRE/ASRM – Sponsored PCOS Consensus Workshop Group. Consensus on infertility treatment related to polycystic ovary syndrome. Human Reprod. 2008; 23: 462-77.

- Tulandi T, Martin J, Al-Fadhli R, et al. Congenital malformations among 911 newborns conceived after infertility treatment with letrozole or clomiphene citrate. Fertil Steril. 2006; 85: 1761-5.

- Tummon I, Gavrilova-Jordan L, Allemand M, et al. Polycystic ovaries and OHSS: a systematic review. Acta Obstet Gynecol Scand. 2005; 84: 611-6.

- Wang J, Davies M, Norman R. PCOS and the risk of spontaneous abortion following ART treatment. Hum Reprod. 2001; 16: 2606-9.

- Wang J, Zhang W, Jiang H, et al. Mutations in HFM1 in recessive primary ovarian insufficiency. N Engl J Med. 2014; 370: 972-4.

- Whelan J, Vlahos N. The ovarian hyperstimulation syndrome. Fertil Steril. 2000; 73: 883-96.

- Wright V, Chang J, Jeng G, et al. ART surveillance - U.S., 2003. MMWR Surveill Summ. 2006; 55: 1-22.

www.ingramcontent.com/pod-product-compliance
Lightning Source LLC
Chambersburg PA
CBHW061159180526
45170CB00002B/879